Created by <u>BabyDreamers.net</u>

Free Book Offer:

Get How to be a Super Mom For Free

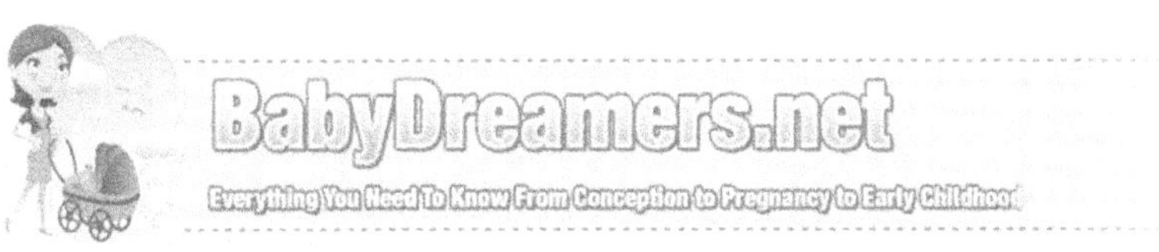

A Short Read is a type of book that is designed to be read in one quick sitting.

These no fluff books are perfect for people who want an overview about a subject in a short period of time.

Table of Contents

The Role of Exercise in Boosting Fertility

The role of exercise in boosting fertility is a topic of great interest for individuals who are trying to conceive. Regular physical activity has been found to have a positive impact on fertility in both men and women. By understanding the link between exercise and fertility, individuals can make informed choices to optimize their chances of conception.

Exercise plays a crucial role in improving hormonal balance, which is essential for fertility. Hormones such as estrogen and progesterone play a key role in regulating the reproductive system. Regular exercise helps to regulate these hormones, creating a more favorable environment for conception.

In addition to hormonal balance, exercise also has a direct effect on ovulation in women. Regular physical activity enhances regular ovulation, increasing the chances of successful conception. For men, exercise can improve sperm health by enhancing sperm quality, motility, and overall reproductive function.

Managing weight and maintaining a healthy body mass index (BMI) is another important aspect of fertility. Obesity has been linked to decreased fertility in both men and women. Exercise helps to manage weight and BMI, reducing the negative impact of obesity on fertility.

Furthermore, exercise has a significant impact on reducing stress and anxiety, which can have a detrimental effect on fertility. Stress has been shown to interfere with reproductive hormones and disrupt the menstrual cycle. By incorporating exercise into their routine, individuals can alleviate stress levels and improve their fertility.

Exercise also enhances blood flow to the reproductive organs, promoting better circulation and improving fertility. Increased blood flow to the pelvic region supports reproductive health and can potentially enhance sexual function and satisfaction.

Moreover, exercise has been found to optimize the quality of eggs and sperm, increasing the likelihood of successful conception. Regular physical activity can enhance egg quality and reduce the risk of chromosomal abnormalities. It also protects sperm DNA from damage, improving fertility outcomes.

The timing and duration of exercise are crucial factors to consider when aiming to boost fertility. Certain types of exercise, such as aerobic activities and strength training, have been found to be particularly effective for improving fertility. It is important to find a balance and avoid excessive exercise, as overtraining can have a negative impact on fertility.

For women with irregular menstrual cycles, exercise can help regulate their cycles and improve fertility. However, women who experience exercise-induced amenorrhea should seek guidance from healthcare professionals to address any potential issues.

When undergoing assisted reproductive technologies (ART) such as in vitro fertilization (IVF) or intrauterine insemination (IUI), exercise can complement these treatments and improve their success rates. However, precautions and guidelines should be followed to ensure safety and effectiveness.

Developing a balanced exercise routine is essential for enhancing fertility. Combining cardiovascular and strength training exercises can provide comprehensive benefits. Rest and recovery periods within the exercise routine are also important for overall fertility health.

It is crucial to consult with a healthcare professional when incorporating exercise for fertility purposes. Individualized exercise recommendations based on specific fertility goals and health conditions are important to ensure optimal outcomes. Monitoring and adjusting exercise intensity is also necessary to optimize fertility results.

In conclusion, exercise plays a significant role in boosting fertility and increasing the chances of successful conception. By understanding the impact of exercise on fertility and following personalized exercise recommendations, individuals can take proactive steps towards improving their fertility health.

The Link Between Exercise and Fertility

The link between exercise and fertility is a topic of growing interest and research. Regular physical activity has been shown to have a positive influence on fertility in both men and women. By engaging in exercise, individuals can potentially improve their chances of conceiving and increase their overall fertility.

Exercise has been found to play a role in various aspects of fertility, including hormonal balance, weight management, stress reduction, blood flow to reproductive organs, and the quality of eggs and sperm. By understanding the connection between exercise and fertility, individuals can make informed decisions about incorporating physical activity into their lifestyle to enhance their reproductive health.

Improving Hormonal Balance

Improving Hormonal Balance

When it comes to fertility, hormonal balance plays a crucial role. Hormones like estrogen and progesterone are essential for regulating the reproductive system and ensuring optimal fertility. Fortunately, exercise can have a positive impact on hormonal balance, helping to regulate these key hormones.

Regular physical activity has been shown to increase the production of endorphins, which are known as "feel-good" hormones. These endorphins can help reduce stress levels, which in turn can have a positive effect on hormone regulation. Stress is known to disrupt the delicate balance of hormones, including estrogen and progesterone, which can interfere with fertility.

Additionally, exercise can help regulate insulin levels in the body. Insulin is a hormone that plays a role in metabolism and can affect reproductive hormones. By maintaining stable insulin levels through exercise, individuals can support hormonal balance and improve their chances of conceiving.

Incorporating aerobic exercises, such as jogging or cycling, into your routine can be particularly beneficial for hormonal regulation. These types of exercises increase heart rate and stimulate the release of hormones that can help regulate estrogen and progesterone levels.

It's important to note that while exercise can have a positive impact on hormonal balance, excessive or intense exercise can have the opposite effect. Overtraining or pushing your body too hard can lead to hormonal imbalances and menstrual irregularities. It's crucial to find a balance and listen to your body's needs when it comes to exercise for fertility.

Effect of Exercise on Ovulation

The effect of exercise on ovulation is a topic of great interest for individuals trying to conceive. Regular physical activity has been shown to enhance regular ovulation, which in turn increases the chances of conception. When we engage in exercise, our body releases endorphins, which are known as "feel-good" hormones. These endorphins can have a positive impact on our reproductive system, promoting regular ovulation.

Exercise also helps to regulate hormone levels, such as estrogen and progesterone, which are essential for fertility. By maintaining a healthy balance of these hormones, exercise can create an optimal environment for conception. Additionally, physical activity can improve blood circulation to the reproductive organs, ensuring that they receive the necessary nutrients and oxygen for optimal function.

It's important to note that excessive exercise or intense workouts can have the opposite effect and disrupt ovulation. Finding the right balance is key. Moderate and regular exercise, such as brisk walking, swimming, or cycling, is generally recommended for enhancing ovulation and fertility. It's always best to consult with a healthcare professional to determine the most suitable exercise routine for your individual needs and fertility goals.

Exercise and Sperm Health

Exercise plays a crucial role in promoting overall reproductive health in men, including the quality and function of sperm. Regular physical activity has been shown to have positive effects on sperm quality, motility, and overall reproductive function. Let's delve into how exercise can benefit sperm health.

Sperm Quality: Exercise has been found to improve sperm quality by increasing antioxidant levels in the body. Antioxidants help protect sperm from oxidative stress, which can damage their DNA and impair their ability to fertilize an egg. By engaging in regular exercise, men can enhance their antioxidant defense system, leading to better sperm quality.

Sperm Motility: Motility refers to the ability of sperm to move effectively towards an egg for fertilization. Exercise has been shown to improve sperm motility by increasing blood flow to the testicles and promoting the production of healthy sperm. Physical activity also helps maintain optimal body temperature, which is essential for sperm production and motility.

Reproductive Function: Exercise can have a positive impact on overall reproductive function in men. It helps regulate hormone levels, including testosterone, which is essential for sperm production. Regular physical activity also improves cardiovascular health, which plays a crucial role in maintaining proper blood flow to the reproductive organs, supporting their optimal function.

Incorporating aerobic exercises, such as running, swimming, or cycling, into your routine can be particularly beneficial for sperm health. These activities increase heart rate and promote better blood circulation throughout the body, including the reproductive system. Strength training exercises, such as weightlifting, can also contribute to improved sperm quality and reproductive function.

It's important to note that excessive exercise and overtraining can have negative effects on sperm health. It's crucial to find a balance and avoid excessive strain on the body. Consulting with a healthcare professional or fertility specialist can provide personalized guidance on the appropriate exercise intensity and duration for optimal sperm health.

Managing Weight and BMI

Managing weight and maintaining a healthy body mass index (BMI) is crucial for optimal fertility. Exercise plays a significant role in achieving and maintaining a healthy weight, which can positively impact fertility outcomes. By engaging in regular physical activity, individuals can effectively manage their weight and BMI, increasing their chances of conceiving.

Exercise helps burn calories and promotes fat loss, which can contribute to achieving a healthy weight. It also helps build lean muscle mass, which can boost metabolism and improve overall body composition. By incorporating a combination of cardiovascular exercises, such as running or cycling, and strength training exercises, like weightlifting or resistance training, individuals can effectively manage their weight and BMI.

In addition to weight management, exercise also helps regulate hormonal balance, which is essential for fertility. Regular physical activity can help regulate the levels of hormones such as estrogen and progesterone, which play a crucial role in reproductive health. By maintaining hormonal balance through exercise, individuals can optimize their fertility potential.

It is important to note that excessive exercise or extreme weight loss can have negative effects on fertility. It is recommended to consult with a healthcare professional or fertility specialist to determine the appropriate exercise regimen and ensure it aligns with individual fertility goals and health conditions. By combining exercise with a healthy diet and lifestyle, individuals can create a balanced approach to managing weight and BMI, ultimately enhancing their fertility.

The Impact of Obesity on Fertility

Obesity can have a significant impact on fertility, affecting both men and women. Excess body weight can disrupt hormonal balance, leading to irregular menstrual cycles in women and decreased sperm quality in men. Additionally, obesity is associated with an increased risk of conditions such as polycystic ovary syndrome (PCOS) and insulin resistance, which can further impair fertility.

In women, obesity can disrupt the delicate balance of hormones necessary for regular ovulation. This can result in irregular or absent menstrual cycles, making it more challenging to conceive. Obesity is also associated with a higher risk of pregnancy complications, such as gestational diabetes and preeclampsia.

For men, obesity can negatively impact sperm quality and reproductive function. Studies have shown that overweight or obese men often have lower sperm counts, decreased sperm motility, and higher rates of DNA damage in sperm. These factors can significantly reduce fertility and increase the risk of infertility.

Fortunately, exercise can play a crucial role in combating the negative effects of obesity on fertility. Regular physical activity can help individuals achieve and maintain a healthy weight, which is essential for optimal reproductive function. Exercise can also improve insulin sensitivity, reducing the risk of conditions like PCOS and insulin resistance.

When combined with a balanced diet, exercise can promote weight loss and improve overall metabolic health. This, in turn, can regulate hormonal balance and enhance fertility. Engaging in regular aerobic exercise, such as brisk walking, swimming, or cycling, can help burn calories and promote weight loss.

Strength training exercises, such as weightlifting or resistance training, can also be beneficial for individuals looking to improve fertility. Building muscle mass can boost metabolism and increase the body's ability to burn calories even at rest. Additionally, strength training can help improve insulin sensitivity and promote hormonal balance.

It's important to note that individuals with obesity-related fertility issues should consult with a healthcare professional before starting an exercise program. A healthcare professional can provide personalized recommendations based on individual needs and goals. They can also help monitor progress and ensure that exercise is safe and effective.

In conclusion, obesity can have a negative impact on fertility in both men and women. However, incorporating regular exercise into a healthy lifestyle can help combat the negative effects of obesity on fertility. By maintaining a healthy weight, improving hormonal balance, and promoting overall reproductive health, exercise can increase the chances of successful conception.

Exercise and Weight Loss

The relationship between exercise, weight loss, and improved fertility outcomes is a topic of great interest for individuals trying to conceive. Research has shown that maintaining a healthy weight is crucial for optimizing fertility in both men and women. Exercise plays a significant role in achieving and maintaining a healthy weight, making it an essential component of any fertility-enhancing plan.

Regular physical activity helps to burn calories and increase metabolism, which can contribute to weight loss. By engaging in exercises that elevate heart rate and promote sweating, individuals can effectively shed excess pounds and reduce body fat. This weight loss can have a positive impact on fertility by improving hormonal balance and enhancing reproductive function.

When individuals are overweight or obese, hormonal imbalances can occur, leading to irregular menstrual cycles in women and reduced sperm quality in men. Exercise can help regulate hormones, such as estrogen and progesterone, which are essential for fertility. By reducing excess weight, exercise can restore hormonal balance and increase the chances of successful conception.

Furthermore, exercise not only aids in weight loss but also improves overall physical and mental well-being. It can reduce stress and anxiety, which are known to have negative effects on fertility. By incorporating exercise into a daily routine, individuals can alleviate stress levels and create a more favorable environment for conception.

It is important to note that exercise should be approached in a balanced and sustainable manner. Extreme or excessive exercise can have the opposite effect on fertility, leading to irregular menstrual cycles or even amenorrhea in women. Therefore, it is crucial to consult with a healthcare professional to determine the appropriate frequency and intensity of exercise for fertility purposes.

In conclusion, exercise and weight loss are closely linked to improved fertility outcomes. By incorporating regular physical activity into one's routine and achieving a healthy weight, individuals can optimize their chances of conceiving. Exercise not only aids in weight loss but also improves hormonal balance, reduces stress, and enhances overall well-being. With the guidance of a healthcare professional, individuals can develop a personalized exercise plan that supports their fertility goals.

Reducing Stress and Anxiety

Exercise not only has physical benefits for fertility, but it also plays a crucial role in reducing stress and anxiety, which can have a positive impact on fertility outcomes. Engaging in regular physical activity has been shown to release endorphins, also known as "feel-good" hormones, which help reduce stress levels and promote a sense of well-being.

When we experience stress, our body releases cortisol, a hormone that can disrupt the delicate balance of reproductive hormones. This can interfere with ovulation and the overall reproductive process. By incorporating exercise into your routine, you can effectively manage stress levels and minimize the negative impact on fertility.

Exercise serves as a healthy outlet for managing the emotional stress that often accompanies the journey of trying to conceive. It allows individuals to channel their energy and emotions in a positive way, providing a sense of control and empowerment. Whether it's going for a run, practicing yoga, or participating in a group fitness class, exercise can help individuals cope with the emotional challenges of infertility.

Furthermore, exercise can also improve sleep quality, which is essential for overall well-being and fertility. Adequate rest and quality sleep are crucial for hormone regulation, including reproductive hormones. By reducing stress and anxiety through exercise, individuals may experience improved sleep patterns, allowing their bodies to function optimally for conception.

Incorporating exercise into your daily routine not only has physical benefits but also offers a multitude of mental and emotional advantages. It can help reduce stress and anxiety, promote a sense of well-being, and improve sleep quality, all of which contribute to a more fertile environment for conception. So, lace up your sneakers and get moving for a healthier body and mind on your fertility journey.

Stress and Fertility

It is well-known that stress can have a significant impact on various aspects of our health, including fertility. When stress levels are high, it can disrupt the delicate balance of hormones in the body, affecting reproductive function and making it more difficult to conceive.

Chronic stress can lead to irregular menstrual cycles, hormonal imbalances, and even ovulation problems. For women, these factors can greatly reduce the chances of getting pregnant. Additionally, stress can also affect sperm production and quality in men, further complicating the fertility journey.

Fortunately, exercise has been shown to be an effective tool in managing and reducing stress levels. Physical activity releases endorphins, which are natural mood boosters that help combat stress and anxiety. By incorporating regular exercise into your routine, you can help alleviate the negative effects of stress on fertility.

Exercise not only provides a distraction from daily worries but also helps to regulate stress hormones such as cortisol. This can have a positive impact on reproductive health by promoting a more balanced hormonal environment. Furthermore, exercise can serve as a healthy coping mechanism, allowing individuals to channel their emotions and frustrations in a productive way.

Whether it's going for a jog, practicing yoga, or engaging in any form of physical activity that you enjoy, finding time for exercise can significantly reduce stress levels and improve your overall well-being. By incorporating exercise into your fertility journey, you are taking a proactive step towards enhancing your chances of conception.

Exercise as a Coping Mechanism

Infertility can be an emotionally challenging journey for individuals and couples alike. The stress and anxiety that often accompany this struggle can take a toll on mental well-being. However, exercise can serve as a valuable coping mechanism, providing a healthy outlet for managing the emotional stress of infertility.

Engaging in regular physical activity releases endorphins, also known as "feel-good" hormones, which can help reduce stress and improve mood. Exercise offers a distraction from the constant thoughts and worries associated with infertility, allowing individuals to focus their energy on something positive and uplifting.

Moreover, exercise provides a sense of control and empowerment. While infertility may feel like a situation beyond one's control, engaging in physical activity allows individuals to take charge of their bodies and overall well-being. It can boost self-esteem and confidence, providing a much-needed sense of accomplishment and empowerment during a challenging time.

Additionally, exercise can help individuals connect with others who may be going through similar experiences. Joining support groups or participating in fitness classes specifically designed for individuals dealing with infertility can create a sense of community and provide a safe space for sharing feelings and experiences.

It's important to note that exercise should be approached with moderation and individualized to one's physical abilities and limitations. Consulting with a healthcare professional or fertility specialist is crucial to ensure that the chosen exercise routine is safe and appropriate for managing the emotional stress of infertility.

In conclusion, exercise can serve as a valuable coping mechanism for individuals facing the emotional stress of infertility. It provides a healthy outlet for managing anxiety, reducing stress levels, and promoting overall well-being. By incorporating regular physical activity into their lives, individuals can find solace, empowerment, and a sense of community during their fertility journey.

Enhancing Blood Flow to the Reproductive Organs

Enhancing Blood Flow to the Reproductive Organs

Exercise plays a crucial role in promoting better blood circulation to the reproductive organs, which in turn can significantly improve fertility. When we engage in physical activity, our heart rate increases, and blood flow is enhanced throughout the body, including the pelvic region where the reproductive organs are located. This increased blood flow delivers vital nutrients and oxygen to the ovaries, uterus, and testes, supporting their optimal function.

Regular exercise helps to dilate blood vessels, allowing for improved circulation and nutrient delivery to the reproductive organs. This can have a positive impact on fertility by enhancing the overall health and vitality of these organs. Furthermore, exercise can also help to reduce inflammation, which can hinder blood flow and impair reproductive function.

It is important to note that different types of exercise can have varying effects on blood flow to the reproductive organs. Aerobic activities, such as jogging, swimming, or cycling, are particularly effective in promoting cardiovascular health and increasing blood circulation. Additionally, strength training exercises, such as weightlifting or resistance training, can also contribute to improved blood flow by strengthening the muscles and improving overall vascular health.

Incorporating exercises that specifically target the pelvic region can further enhance blood flow to the reproductive organs. Pelvic floor exercises, such as Kegels, can help strengthen the pelvic muscles and improve blood circulation in this area. Yoga and Pilates are also beneficial for promoting blood flow to the reproductive organs, as they focus on stretching and strengthening the pelvic area.

By engaging in regular exercise that promotes better blood flow to the reproductive organs, individuals can increase their chances of achieving successful conception. It is important to consult with a healthcare professional to determine the most suitable exercise routine based on individual needs and fertility goals.

Exercise and Pelvic Blood Flow

Exercise plays a crucial role in promoting reproductive health by increasing blood flow to the pelvic region. Physical activity stimulates the cardiovascular system, causing blood vessels to dilate and allowing for better circulation throughout the body. When it comes to fertility, improved blood flow to the pelvic area is particularly beneficial as it supports the health and function of the reproductive organs.

Increasing blood flow to the pelvic region through exercise can have several positive effects on reproductive health. Firstly, it helps to nourish the ovaries and uterus, providing them with essential nutrients and oxygen. This can enhance the overall health of these organs and improve their ability to function optimally.

In addition, exercise-induced blood flow to the pelvic region can aid in the removal of toxins and waste products from the reproductive organs. This cleansing effect can contribute to a healthier reproductive environment, increasing the chances of successful conception.

Furthermore, improved blood flow to the pelvic area can also support hormonal balance, which is crucial for fertility. Hormones play a vital role in regulating the menstrual cycle and ovulation. By promoting better blood circulation, exercise can help ensure that hormones reach their intended targets in a timely manner, facilitating regular ovulation and optimizing fertility.

It is worth noting that different types of exercise can have varying effects on pelvic blood flow. Aerobic activities, such as jogging, swimming, or cycling, are particularly effective in increasing blood circulation throughout the body, including the pelvic region. Strength training exercises, on the other hand, may not have as direct of an impact on pelvic blood flow but can still contribute to overall cardiovascular health, which indirectly supports reproductive function.

It is important to note that while exercise can be beneficial for pelvic blood flow and reproductive health, moderation is key. Overexertion or intense exercise regimens may have the opposite effect, leading to decreased blood flow to the pelvic region. It is always recommended to consult with a healthcare professional before starting any new exercise routine, especially if you are trying to conceive or have any underlying health conditions.

Improving Sexual Function

Improving Sexual Function

Regular exercise has been shown to have a positive impact on sexual function and satisfaction, which can potentially increase fertility. Engaging in physical activity can improve overall cardiovascular health, increase blood flow to the pelvic region, and enhance sexual arousal and performance.

When we exercise, our bodies release endorphins, also known as "feel-good" hormones, which can boost mood and reduce stress. This can have a direct impact on sexual desire and pleasure. Additionally, exercise can help improve body image and self-confidence, which are important factors in sexual satisfaction.

Incorporating aerobic exercises, such as running, swimming, or cycling, into your routine can help improve stamina and endurance, allowing for longer and more enjoyable sexual experiences. Strength training exercises, on the other hand, can enhance muscle tone and strength, which can lead to increased sexual pleasure for both partners.

It's important to note that the benefits of exercise on sexual function may vary from person to person. It's always best to consult with a healthcare professional to determine the most suitable exercise routine for your individual needs and goals.

Optimizing Egg and Sperm Quality

The quality of eggs and sperm plays a crucial role in the success of conception. Fortunately, exercise can have a positive impact on optimizing the quality of both eggs and sperm, increasing the chances of successful fertility outcomes.

For women, regular exercise has been shown to enhance egg quality and reduce the risk of chromosomal abnormalities. This is particularly important as women age and their egg quality naturally declines. Exercise can help improve blood flow to the ovaries, providing the necessary nutrients and oxygen for the development of healthy eggs. Additionally, physical activity can stimulate the production of antioxidants, which protect the eggs from oxidative stress and damage.

Similarly, exercise can benefit sperm quality in men. Studies have demonstrated that active men tend to have higher sperm counts, better motility, and lower levels of DNA damage in their sperm. Physical activity can improve blood flow to the testes, promoting the production of healthier sperm. Furthermore, exercise can help regulate hormone levels in men, such as testosterone, which is essential for sperm production and function.

Incorporating regular exercise into your routine can be a proactive step in optimizing the quality of eggs and sperm, ultimately increasing the likelihood of successful conception. Remember to consult with a healthcare professional to receive personalized exercise recommendations based on your individual fertility goals and health conditions.

Exercise and Egg Quality

Exercise plays a crucial role in enhancing egg quality and reducing the risk of chromosomal abnormalities. Regular physical activity can have a positive impact on fertility by improving overall reproductive health. When it comes to egg quality, exercise has been found to stimulate the production of antioxidants, which help protect the eggs from damage and improve their quality.

Furthermore, exercise promotes better blood circulation to the ovaries, ensuring that the eggs receive an adequate supply of oxygen and nutrients. This improved blood flow also helps remove toxins and waste products from the reproductive organs, creating a healthier environment for egg development.

Studies have shown that women who engage in moderate-intensity exercise, such as brisk walking or cycling, have a higher chance of producing high-quality eggs. Exercise not only enhances egg quality but also reduces the risk of chromosomal abnormalities, which can lead to miscarriages or genetic disorders in the offspring.

It's important to note that excessive exercise or intense training can have the opposite effect on egg quality. Overexertion and extreme physical stress can disrupt hormonal balance and negatively impact fertility. Therefore, it's crucial to find a balance and engage in moderate exercise that supports reproductive health without causing excessive strain.

Incorporating a variety of exercises, such as aerobic activities, strength training, and yoga, can provide comprehensive benefits for egg quality. Aerobic exercises increase heart rate and improve overall cardiovascular health, while strength training helps build muscle strength and improve metabolism. Yoga and other mind-body exercises can help reduce stress levels and promote relaxation, which is essential for optimal fertility.

Consulting with a healthcare professional or fertility specialist is recommended before starting any exercise routine, especially for individuals with pre-existing health conditions or specific fertility concerns. They can provide personalized exercise recommendations based on individual needs and goals, ensuring that the exercise routine is safe and effective.

Exercise and Sperm DNA Integrity

Exercise and Sperm DNA Integrity

Physical activity plays a crucial role in protecting sperm DNA integrity, which in turn can have a positive impact on fertility outcomes. Sperm DNA integrity refers to the quality and stability of the genetic material within sperm cells. When sperm DNA is damaged or fragmented, it can lead to reduced fertility and an increased risk of miscarriage.

Regular exercise has been shown to improve sperm DNA integrity by reducing oxidative stress and inflammation in the reproductive system. Oxidative stress occurs when there is an imbalance between the production of reactive oxygen species (ROS) and the body's ability to neutralize them.

High levels of ROS can cause damage to sperm DNA, leading to fertility issues.

Exercise helps to combat oxidative stress by increasing antioxidant defenses in the body. Antioxidants are molecules that neutralize ROS and protect sperm DNA from damage. Additionally, physical activity improves blood flow to the testes, providing essential nutrients and oxygen to support healthy sperm production and function.

It's important to note that excessive exercise or intense training can have the opposite effect and actually increase oxidative stress, potentially harming sperm DNA integrity. Therefore, it's crucial to strike a balance and engage in moderate exercise that supports overall health without overexertion.

Exercise Recommendations for Sperm DNA Integrity

When it comes to exercise for improving sperm DNA integrity, it's recommended to focus on moderate-intensity activities such as brisk walking, jogging, swimming, or cycling. These aerobic exercises help increase blood flow to the reproductive organs, including the testes, promoting better sperm quality and DNA integrity.

Incorporating strength training exercises, such as weightlifting or resistance band workouts, can also be beneficial. Strength training helps build muscle mass and improve overall fitness, which can positively impact sperm health and DNA integrity.

It's important to consult with a healthcare professional or fertility specialist before starting any exercise regimen, especially if you have existing fertility concerns. They can provide personalized recommendations based on your individual needs and help monitor your progress.

Remember, exercise is just one piece of the puzzle when it comes to optimizing fertility. It should be combined with a healthy diet, stress management techniques, and other lifestyle factors to maximize your chances of conception and a healthy pregnancy.

Timing and Duration of Exercise

The timing and duration of exercise play a crucial role in enhancing fertility. It is important to understand the optimal timing and duration of exercise to maximize its benefits for fertility enhancement. By following the right timing and duration, individuals can increase their chances of conceiving and improve overall reproductive health.

When it comes to timing, it is recommended to engage in regular exercise throughout the week. Consistency is key, as sporadic or irregular exercise may not yield the desired results. Allocating specific time slots for exercise and sticking to a routine can help establish a healthy exercise habit.

Additionally, it is important to consider the duration of exercise sessions. While the exact duration may vary depending on individual fitness levels and goals, it is generally recommended to aim for at least 150 minutes of moderate-intensity exercise or 75 minutes of vigorous-intensity exercise per week. This can be further divided into smaller sessions throughout the week to ensure regular physical activity.

It is worth noting that exercise intensity should be tailored to individual capabilities and preferences. It is important to find a balance between challenging oneself and avoiding excessive strain or exhaustion. Consulting with a healthcare professional or a certified fitness trainer can provide personalized guidance on the appropriate timing, duration, and intensity of exercise for fertility enhancement.

The Best Types of Exercise for Fertility

The best types of exercise for improving fertility include aerobic activities and strength training. Aerobic exercises, such as running, swimming, and cycling, are known to increase heart rate and improve cardiovascular health. These exercises help in maintaining a healthy weight and body mass index (BMI), which are crucial factors for optimal fertility.

Strength training exercises, on the other hand, focus on building muscle strength and improving overall body composition. Resistance training, using weights or resistance bands, can help increase muscle mass and boost metabolism. This can contribute to better hormonal balance and enhance fertility outcomes.

It is important to note that finding a balance between aerobic activities and strength training is key. Combining both types of exercises in a well-rounded routine can provide maximum benefits for fertility. This can be achieved by alternating between cardio sessions and strength training sessions throughout the week.

Additionally, incorporating flexibility exercises, such as yoga or Pilates, can help improve overall body flexibility and reduce muscle tension. These exercises can also promote relaxation and reduce stress, which are important factors for fertility.

Overall, a combination of aerobic activities, strength training, and flexibility exercises can be considered the best types of exercise for improving fertility. It is important to consult with a healthcare professional or fertility specialist to develop a personalized exercise plan that suits individual needs and goals.

Exercise Frequency and Duration

When it comes to exercise for optimal fertility benefits, both frequency and duration play a crucial role. The recommended frequency of exercise is typically around 3-5 times per week. This allows for consistent physical activity without overexertion. It's important to find a balance that works for your body and schedule.

In terms of duration, aim for at least 30 minutes of moderate-intensity exercise per session. This can include activities such as brisk walking, cycling, or swimming. However, it's important to note that longer durations or higher intensity workouts may not necessarily lead to better fertility outcomes. Overdoing exercise can actually have a negative impact on fertility, so it's important to listen to your body and not push yourself too hard.

Additionally, it's beneficial to incorporate a variety of exercises into your routine. This can include both cardiovascular exercises, such as jogging or dancing, and strength training exercises, such as weightlifting or yoga. This combination helps to improve overall fitness and support reproductive health.

Remember, every individual is unique, and what works for one person may not work for another. It's always a good idea to consult with a healthcare professional or fertility specialist to get personalized exercise recommendations based on your specific fertility goals and health conditions. They can provide guidance on the ideal frequency and duration of exercise that will optimize your fertility outcomes.

Considerations for Women with Irregular Cycles

Addressing the unique considerations and challenges for women with irregular menstrual cycles is crucial when discussing the role of exercise in boosting fertility. Irregular cycles can make it difficult to track ovulation and determine the most fertile days for conception. However, exercise can play a significant role in regulating menstrual cycles and improving fertility outcomes.

For women with irregular cycles, it is important to consult with a healthcare professional before starting an exercise routine. They can provide personalized recommendations based on individual health conditions and fertility goals. In some cases, certain exercises may need to be modified or avoided to prevent further disruption to the menstrual cycle.

Incorporating aerobic activities, such as walking, jogging, or cycling, can help regulate hormone levels and promote regular ovulation. These exercises increase blood flow to the reproductive organs, supporting overall reproductive health. Strength training exercises, like weightlifting or yoga, can also be beneficial for women with irregular cycles by improving hormonal balance and reducing stress levels.

Additionally, maintaining a healthy body weight through exercise and a balanced diet is essential for women with irregular cycles. Excess body weight or rapid weight loss can contribute to hormonal imbalances and irregular periods. Therefore, a combination of cardiovascular exercises and strength training, along with a focus on maintaining a healthy weight, can help regulate menstrual cycles and improve fertility outcomes for women with irregular cycles.

Exercise and Menstrual Irregularities

Menstrual irregularities can be a frustrating and challenging issue for women trying to conceive. However, incorporating regular exercise into your routine can have a positive impact on regulating menstrual cycles and improving fertility in women with irregular periods.

Exercise helps to balance hormones, such as estrogen and progesterone, which play a crucial role in the menstrual cycle. By engaging in physical activity, you can stimulate the release of these hormones, promoting a more regular menstrual cycle and increasing the chances of ovulation.

In addition to hormonal regulation, exercise also improves blood circulation to the reproductive organs, including the uterus. This increased blood flow can help nourish the uterine lining, making it more receptive to implantation and increasing the chances of successful conception.

It is important to note that while exercise can be beneficial for women with irregular periods, it is essential to find the right balance. Intense or excessive exercise can have the opposite effect and disrupt the menstrual cycle further. Therefore, it is recommended to consult with a healthcare professional to determine the appropriate level and type of exercise for your specific situation.

By incorporating regular exercise into your routine, you can help regulate your menstrual cycle, improve fertility, and increase your chances of conceiving.

Overcoming Exercise-Related Amenorrhea

Overcoming Exercise-Related Amenorrhea

Exercise-induced amenorrhea is a condition where women experience the absence of menstrual periods due to excessive physical activity. This can have a significant impact on fertility, as regular menstrual cycles are essential for ovulation and conception. However, there are strategies that women can implement to overcome exercise-related amenorrhea and improve their chances of becoming pregnant.

Firstly, it is crucial to reassess the intensity and duration of your exercise routine. High-intensity workouts and excessive training can disrupt hormonal balance and suppress the release of reproductive hormones necessary for ovulation. Consider reducing the intensity and duration of your workouts to allow your body to recover and restore hormonal balance.

Incorporating rest days into your exercise routine is also essential. Rest days provide your body with the opportunity to recover and reduce stress levels. Overtraining and chronic stress can negatively impact fertility by disrupting the delicate hormonal balance needed for regular menstrual cycles. Prioritize rest and recovery to support your reproductive health.

Additionally, it may be beneficial to include more low-impact exercises in your routine, such as yoga or swimming. These activities can help reduce the physical stress on your body while still providing the benefits of regular exercise. Low-impact exercises can also help regulate hormone levels and promote regular menstrual cycles.

Furthermore, maintaining a balanced and nutritious diet is crucial for overcoming exercise-related amenorrhea. Ensure you are consuming enough calories and nutrients to support your body's energy needs. Adequate nutrition is essential for hormone production and overall reproductive health.

Lastly, it is important to consult with a healthcare professional who specializes in fertility and exercise. They can provide personalized recommendations and guidance based on your individual needs and goals. They can also monitor your progress and make necessary adjustments to your exercise routine to optimize fertility outcomes.

Remember, overcoming exercise-induced amenorrhea requires a holistic approach that includes modifying your exercise routine, prioritizing rest and recovery, maintaining a balanced diet, and seeking professional guidance. By taking these steps, you can restore hormonal balance, regulate menstrual cycles, and improve your chances of achieving a healthy pregnancy.

Exercise and Assisted Reproductive Technologies (ART)

Exercise can play a significant role in conjunction with Assisted Reproductive Technologies (ART), such as in vitro fertilization (IVF) or intrauterine insemination (IUI). These fertility treatments can be physically and emotionally demanding, and exercise can help support their effectiveness and improve overall outcomes.

When undergoing ART, it is essential to consult with a healthcare professional to determine the most appropriate exercise routine for your specific situation. They can provide personalized recommendations based on your fertility goals and health conditions.

While exercise is generally beneficial for fertility, it is crucial to be mindful of certain precautions during ART. High-impact exercises or activities that put excessive strain on the body should be avoided to prevent any potential harm or complications. It is recommended to focus on low-impact exercises that promote cardiovascular health and strength training exercises that target major muscle groups.

Additionally, it is important to listen to your body and adjust the intensity of your exercise routine as needed. Overexertion or excessive fatigue can negatively impact fertility outcomes, so it is essential to find the right balance between physical activity and rest.

By incorporating exercise into your routine during ART, you can support the effectiveness of these treatments and enhance your overall fertility health. However, always remember to consult with a healthcare professional to ensure that your exercise routine is safe and suitable for your specific situation.

Optimizing Fertility Treatments

When it comes to fertility treatments, exercise can play a crucial role in enhancing their effectiveness and improving success rates. While fertility treatments like in vitro fertilization (IVF) or intrauterine insemination (IUI) are often the go-to options for couples struggling to conceive, incorporating exercise into the treatment plan can offer additional benefits.

Exercise can complement fertility treatments by improving overall reproductive health, increasing blood flow to the reproductive organs, and regulating hormones. By engaging in regular physical activity, individuals can optimize their fertility treatments and increase their chances of successful conception.

One way exercise can enhance fertility treatments is by improving blood circulation to the reproductive organs. Physical activity promotes better blood flow, ensuring that the reproductive organs receive the necessary nutrients and oxygen for optimal functioning. This improved blood flow can enhance the effectiveness of fertility treatments and create a more conducive environment for conception.

In addition to improving blood flow, exercise can also help regulate hormones, such as estrogen and progesterone, which are essential for fertility. Hormonal balance is crucial during fertility treatments, and exercise can contribute to achieving and maintaining this balance. By engaging in regular exercise, individuals can support their fertility treatments and enhance their chances of a successful outcome.

Furthermore, exercise can also have a positive impact on emotional well-being during fertility treatments. The process of trying to conceive can be emotionally challenging, and exercise can serve as a healthy coping mechanism. Physical activity releases endorphins, which are known as "feel-good" hormones, and can help reduce stress and anxiety associated with fertility treatments.

It is important to note that exercise should be approached with caution during fertility treatments, as certain activities may need to be modified or avoided to ensure the safety and effectiveness of the treatment. Consulting with a healthcare professional or fertility specialist is essential to receive personalized exercise recommendations that align with individual fertility goals and health conditions.

In conclusion, exercise can complement fertility treatments and improve their success rates. By incorporating regular physical activity into the treatment plan, individuals can enhance blood flow to the reproductive organs, regulate hormones, and manage emotional stress. However, it is crucial to seek guidance from a healthcare professional to ensure that exercise is tailored to individual needs and to monitor and adjust exercise intensity for optimal fertility outcomes.

Exercise Precautions during ART

When undergoing fertility treatments such as assisted reproductive technologies (ART), it's important to take certain precautions and follow guidelines to ensure the safety and effectiveness of exercise. While exercise can be beneficial for overall health and fertility, it's essential to tailor your exercise routine to your specific treatment plan and individual needs.

Here are some precautions and guidelines to keep in mind when exercising during ART:

- Consult with your healthcare professional: Before starting or modifying your exercise routine, it's crucial to consult with your healthcare professional, such as your fertility specialist or reproductive endocrinologist. They can provide personalized recommendations based on your specific fertility goals and health conditions.
- Consider the stage of your treatment: The type and intensity of exercise may need to be adjusted depending on the stage of your fertility treatment. For example, during the stimulation phase of in vitro fertilization (IVF), high-impact exercises or activities that put excessive strain on the pelvic area may need to be avoided.
- Listen to your body: Pay attention to how your body responds to exercise during fertility treatments. If you experience any discomfort, pain, or unusual symptoms, it's important to stop exercising and consult with your healthcare professional.
- Avoid excessive heat exposure: High temperatures, such as those in hot tubs, saunas, or hot yoga classes, can negatively impact sperm and egg quality. It's best to avoid prolonged exposure to excessive heat during fertility treatments.

- Choose low-impact exercises: Opt for low-impact exercises that are gentle on the body, such as walking, swimming, prenatal yoga, or stationary cycling. These exercises can help maintain fitness levels without putting excessive strain on the reproductive organs.
- Practice moderation: While regular exercise is important, it's crucial to avoid overexertion or excessive intensity. Strive for a moderate exercise routine that allows for adequate rest and recovery.

Remember, every individual and fertility treatment plan is unique, so it's essential to consult with your healthcare professional for personalized exercise recommendations and guidelines. By taking precautions and following the appropriate guidelines, you can safely incorporate exercise into your fertility journey and optimize your chances of success.

Creating a Balanced Exercise Routine

When it comes to enhancing fertility through exercise, it's important to create a balanced exercise routine that incorporates a variety of activities. By diversifying your workouts, you can target different muscle groups, improve overall fitness, and optimize fertility outcomes. Here are some practical tips for developing a well-rounded exercise routine:

- **Combine Cardiovascular and Strength Training:** Incorporate both aerobic exercises, such as running or cycling, and strength training exercises, like weightlifting or Pilates. Cardiovascular exercises improve heart health and increase blood flow to the reproductive organs, while strength training helps build muscle and support overall body function.
- **Include Flexibility and Stretching:** Don't forget to incorporate flexibility exercises, such as yoga or stretching, into your routine. These activities can improve posture, reduce muscle tension, and enhance overall body flexibility.
- **Alternate High and Low-Intensity Workouts:** Vary the intensity of your workouts by alternating between high-intensity exercises, like interval training or HIIT, and low-intensity activities, such as walking or gentle yoga. This approach helps challenge your body while also allowing for adequate recovery.
- **Listen to Your Body:** Pay attention to how your body feels during and after exercise. If you experience pain or discomfort, modify your routine or consult with a healthcare professional. It's important to find the right balance between pushing yourself and avoiding overexertion.

- **Include Rest and Recovery Days:** Give your body time to rest and recover between workouts. Rest days are just as important as exercise days, as they allow your muscles to repair and rebuild. Aim for at least one or two rest days per week.

Remember, developing a balanced exercise routine is not only beneficial for fertility but also for overall health and well-being. By incorporating a variety of exercises and listening to your body's needs, you can create a routine that supports your fertility goals while promoting overall fitness.

Combining Cardiovascular and Strength Training

Combining cardiovascular and strength training exercises can have numerous benefits for fertility. By incorporating both types of exercises into your routine, you can optimize your chances of conceiving and improve overall reproductive health.

Cardiovascular exercises, such as running, swimming, or cycling, help to improve cardiovascular health and increase blood flow throughout the body, including the reproductive organs. This increased blood flow can enhance the delivery of oxygen and nutrients to the ovaries and uterus, promoting better reproductive function. Additionally, cardiovascular exercises can help to maintain a healthy weight and body mass index (BMI), which are important factors for fertility.

On the other hand, strength training exercises, such as weightlifting or resistance training, can help to build muscle strength and improve overall body composition. By increasing muscle mass, strength training exercises can enhance metabolic function and hormone regulation, including the hormones that play a crucial role in fertility, such as estrogen and progesterone. Strength training exercises can also help to improve bone density, which is important for women's reproductive health.

By combining cardiovascular and strength training exercises, you can reap the benefits of both types of exercises and create a well-rounded fitness routine that supports fertility. It is important to consult with a healthcare professional or a certified fitness trainer to develop an exercise plan tailored to your individual needs and goals. They can provide guidance on the appropriate intensity, duration, and frequency of cardiovascular and strength training exercises to optimize fertility outcomes.

Importance of Rest and Recovery

The importance of rest and recovery cannot be overstated when it comes to maintaining overall fertility health. While exercise is beneficial for boosting fertility, it is equally important to allow the body time to rest and recover between workouts. Rest and recovery periods within an exercise routine play a crucial role in optimizing fertility outcomes.

Rest allows the body to repair and rebuild tissues that have been stressed during exercise. It also helps prevent overtraining, which can have negative effects on fertility. Overtraining can disrupt hormonal balance, interfere with ovulation, and decrease sperm quality. Therefore, incorporating rest days into an exercise routine is essential for maintaining fertility health.

During rest and recovery periods, the body also replenishes energy stores and reduces inflammation. This is especially important for individuals trying to conceive, as inflammation can adversely affect reproductive health. By allowing the body to rest and recover, inflammation levels can be kept in check, promoting optimal fertility.

In addition to rest days, it is important to prioritize sleep as part of the rest and recovery process. Sleep plays a crucial role in hormone regulation, including those involved in fertility. Lack of sleep or poor sleep quality can disrupt hormonal balance, leading to fertility issues. Therefore, ensuring an adequate amount of sleep each night is vital for overall fertility health.

When designing an exercise routine for fertility, it is important to strike a balance between physical activity and rest. Aim for a combination of cardiovascular exercises, strength training, and rest days to optimize fertility outcomes. Consulting with a healthcare professional can provide personalized recommendations based on individual fertility goals and health conditions.

Consulting with a Healthcare Professional

When it comes to incorporating exercise into your fertility journey, it is crucial to consult with a healthcare professional. Seeking guidance from a qualified expert can provide you with personalized recommendations based on your individual fertility goals and health conditions.

A healthcare professional, such as a fertility specialist or reproductive endocrinologist, can assess your specific needs and create an exercise plan tailored to your unique circumstances. They can take into account factors such as your current fitness level, any underlying medical conditions, and the type of fertility treatments you may be undergoing.

By working closely with a healthcare professional, you can ensure that your exercise routine is safe and effective for your fertility goals. They can provide valuable insights into the best types of exercise to incorporate, the ideal frequency and duration of workouts, and any precautions you should take during fertility treatments.

Additionally, a healthcare professional can monitor your progress and adjust your exercise intensity as needed. This ongoing guidance can help optimize your fertility outcomes and ensure that you are on the right track towards achieving your goals.

Remember, fertility is a complex and individualized journey, and seeking professional advice is essential to ensure that your exercise routine aligns with your specific needs. So, don't hesitate to reach out to a healthcare professional who specializes in fertility to get the guidance and support you need.

Individualized Exercise Recommendations

When it comes to boosting fertility through exercise, there is no one-size-fits-all approach. Each individual has unique fertility goals and health conditions that should be taken into consideration when creating an exercise routine. This is why personalized exercise recommendations are crucial for optimizing fertility outcomes.

Consulting with a healthcare professional who specializes in fertility can provide valuable insights into the specific exercise regimen that would be most beneficial for you. They can take into account factors such as your current fitness level, any underlying health conditions, and your fertility goals.

Based on this information, they can recommend exercises that are safe and effective for you. For example, if you are trying to regulate your menstrual cycle, they may suggest incorporating aerobic activities like brisk walking or swimming. If you are looking to improve sperm quality, they may recommend strength training exercises.

In addition to personalized exercise recommendations, your healthcare professional can also guide you on the frequency and duration of your workouts. They can help you strike the right balance between challenging yourself and avoiding overexertion, which can have negative effects on fertility.

Remember, fertility is a complex and individualized journey, and exercise is just one piece of the puzzle. By seeking personalized exercise recommendations, you can ensure that you are taking the right steps towards optimizing your fertility and increasing your chances of conceiving.

Monitoring and Adjusting Exercise Intensity

When it comes to exercise for fertility, it's not just about the type and duration of workouts. Monitoring and adjusting exercise intensity is equally important for optimizing fertility outcomes. By understanding the impact of exercise intensity on the body, individuals can tailor their workouts to enhance their chances of conception.

Monitoring exercise intensity involves paying attention to factors such as heart rate, perceived exertion, and breathing rate during physical activity. These indicators can help individuals gauge the intensity of their workouts and ensure they are within a safe and effective range for fertility benefits.

Adjusting exercise intensity is crucial because what may be appropriate for one person may not be suitable for another. It's essential to listen to your body and make adjustments based on your fitness level, overall health, and fertility goals. Consulting with a healthcare professional or a fertility specialist can provide valuable guidance in determining the optimal exercise intensity for your specific needs.

One way to monitor exercise intensity is by tracking heart rate. The target heart rate zone for fertility-enhancing workouts is typically around 60-80% of your maximum heart rate. This range ensures that you are working hard enough to reap the benefits of exercise without overexerting yourself.

Perceived exertion is another useful tool for monitoring exercise intensity. This involves assessing how hard you feel you are working during a workout on a scale of 1 to 10, with 1 being very light and 10 being maximum effort. Aim for a perceived exertion level of around 6-8 during fertility-focused exercises.

Additionally, paying attention to your breathing rate can provide insights into exercise intensity. If you find it challenging to carry on a conversation while exercising, it may be an indication that the intensity is too high. On the other hand, if you can easily chat without feeling breathless, you may need to increase the intensity to optimize fertility benefits.

Remember, everyone's exercise capacity and fertility goals are unique, so it's essential to personalize your exercise routine accordingly. By monitoring and adjusting exercise intensity, you can ensure that you are maximizing the fertility-enhancing effects of physical activity and increasing your chances of successful conception.

Frequently Asked Questions

- **How does exercise impact fertility?**

Regular exercise can have a positive influence on fertility in both men and women. It helps regulate hormones, improves ovulation, enhances sperm health, manages weight and BMI, reduces stress and anxiety, promotes better blood flow to reproductive organs, and optimizes egg and sperm quality.

- **Can exercise help regulate hormones necessary for fertility?**

Yes, exercise plays a crucial role in regulating hormones such as estrogen and progesterone, which are essential for fertility. Regular physical activity helps maintain a hormonal balance, increasing the chances of successful conception.

- **Does exercise improve ovulation?**

Absolutely! Exercise can enhance regular ovulation, making it easier for women to conceive. By incorporating physical activity into your routine, you can increase the likelihood of successful ovulation and increase your chances of getting pregnant.

- **How does exercise impact sperm health?**

Physical activity has a positive impact on sperm health. It improves sperm quality, motility, and overall reproductive function in men. By engaging in regular exercise, men can increase their fertility potential and improve their chances of successful conception.

- **Can exercise help combat obesity and improve fertility?**

Exercise plays a crucial role in managing weight and body mass index (BMI), which are important factors for fertility. Obesity can negatively affect fertility, but through regular exercise, individuals can combat obesity and improve their chances of conceiving.

- **How does exercise reduce stress and anxiety related to fertility?**

Exercise has stress-reducing benefits and can help alleviate stress and anxiety related to fertility. Physical activity releases endorphins, which are known as "feel-good" hormones, helping individuals manage the emotional stress of infertility and promoting overall well-being.

- **Does exercise improve blood flow to reproductive organs?**

Yes, exercise promotes better blood circulation to the reproductive organs, enhancing fertility. By engaging in physical activity, you can increase blood flow to the pelvic region, supporting reproductive health and improving your chances of conception.

- **Can exercise enhance sexual function and satisfaction?**

Exercise has been shown to enhance sexual function and satisfaction, potentially increasing fertility. By incorporating regular physical activity into your routine, you can improve sexual health, which can positively impact your fertility journey.

- **How does exercise optimize egg and sperm quality?**

Exercise plays a role in improving the quality of eggs and sperm, increasing the likelihood of successful conception. It can enhance egg quality, reduce the risk of chromosomal abnormalities, and protect sperm DNA from damage, ultimately improving fertility outcomes.

- **What are the recommended types and duration of exercise for fertility?**

Aerobic activities and strength training are considered the most effective forms of exercise for improving fertility. It is recommended to engage in moderate-intensity exercise for at least 150 minutes per week, or as advised by a healthcare professional.

- **Can exercise help regulate menstrual cycles for women with irregular periods?**

Yes, exercise can help regulate menstrual cycles and improve fertility in women with irregular periods. By incorporating regular physical activity into their routine, women can promote hormonal balance and increase their chances of successful conception.

- **How does exercise complement fertility treatments like IVF or IUI?**

Exercise can complement fertility treatments such as in vitro fertilization (IVF) or intrauterine insemination (IUI). It can optimize the effectiveness of these treatments and improve success rates. However, it is important to follow precautions and guidelines provided by healthcare professionals.

- **What should be considered when developing a balanced exercise routine for fertility?**

When developing a balanced exercise routine for fertility, it is important to combine cardiovascular and strength training exercises. Rest and recovery periods are also crucial for overall fertility health. Seeking guidance from a healthcare professional is recommended to ensure personalized recommendations.

- **Why is it important to consult with a healthcare professional regarding exercise for fertility?**

Consulting with a healthcare professional is crucial when incorporating exercise for fertility purposes. They can provide individualized exercise recommendations based on specific fertility goals and health conditions. Monitoring and adjusting exercise intensity is essential for optimizing fertility outcomes.

-57-

Have Questions / Comments?

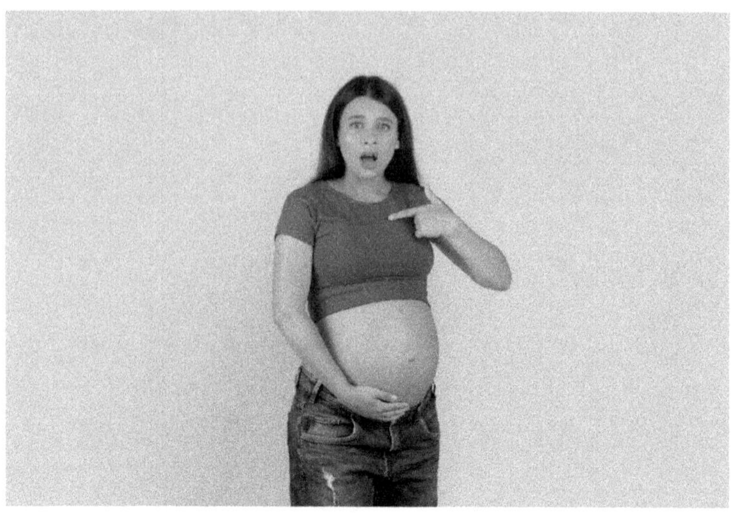

This book was designed to cover as much info as possible but I know I have probably missed something, or some new amazing discovery that has just come out.

If you notice something missing or have a question that I failed to answer, please get in touch and let me know. If I can, I will email you an answer and also update the book so others can also benefit from it.

Thanks For Being Awesome :)

Submit Your Questions / Comments At:

Get In Touch at Babydreamers.net

Get How To Be A Super Mom - 100% FREE

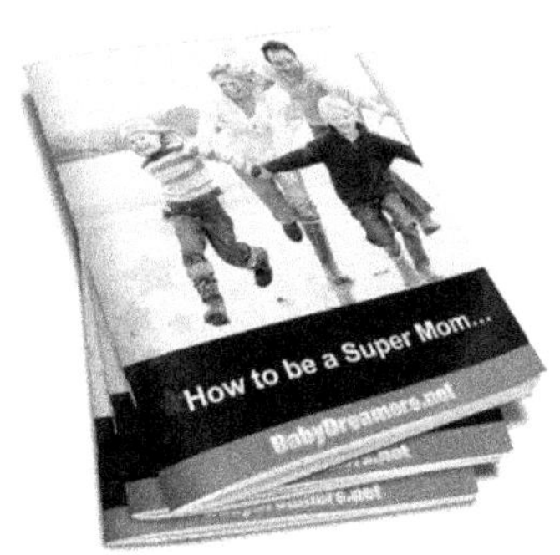

For being one of our amazing readers, we would love to offer you another book we have created, 100% free.

Being a mom is probably the most important job in the world – we've all heard that, and it's true. You're bringing up the next generation of wonderful, intelligent, loving, creative, responsible people.

We all want to be Super Mom and to be everything and do everything, but it this possible?

Being a Super Mom is possible, but you have to learn how to empower yourself to be the kind of Super Mom that you feel you need to be, keeping in mind that the title Super Mom doesn't mean the same thing to everyone.

Get How to be a Super Mom For Free at

BabyDreamers.net